LIFE STYLE WEIGHT MANAGEMENT

DAILY FOOD DAIRY

Date: ………………….

Time you woke up: …………………………………………..

Time you went to bed: ……………………………………………

Please list the brand names, ingredients and portion of each food you eat daily.

Time	Food/Beverages/Ingredients	Portion/Size	Est. Calories	Feel Full?
	Total Calories for the Day			

Describe your activity today:

………

………

………

LIFE STYLE WEIGHT MANAGEMENT

DAILY FOOD DAIRY

Date: …………………….

Time you woke up: ……………………………………………..

Time you went to bed: ……………………………………………

Time	Food/Beverages/Ingredients	Portion/Size	Est. Calories	Feel Full?
	Total Calories for the Day			

Describe your activity today:

………

………

……

LIFE STYLE WEIGHT MANAGEMENT

DAILY FOOD DAIRY

Date: ………………….

Time you woke up: ……………………………………….

Time you went to bed: ……………………………………

Time	Food/Beverages/Ingredients	Portion/Size	Est. Calories	Feel Full?
	Total Calories for the Day			

Describe your activity today:

……

……

……

LIFE STYLE WEIGHT MANAGEMENT

DAILY FOOD DAIRY

Date: …………………

Time you woke up: ……………………………………..

Time you went to bed: …………………………………………

Time	Food/Beverages/Ingredients	Portion/Size	Est. Calories	Feel Full?
	Total Calories for the Day			

Describe your activity today:

……

……

……

DAILY FOOD DAIRY

Date: …………………….

Time you woke up: ………………………………………….

Time you went to bed: …………………………………………….

Please list the brand names, ingredients and portion of each food you eat daily.

Time	Food/Beverages/Ingredients	Portion/Size	Est. Calories	Feel Full?
	Total Calories for the Day			

Describe your activity today:

……

……

………

DAILY FOOD DAIRY

Date: …………………

Time you woke up: ………………………………………..

Time you went to bed: ………………………………………

| Please list the brand names, ingredients and portion of each food you eat daily. |

Time	Food/Beverages/Ingredients	Portion/Size	Est. Calories	Feel Full?
	Total Calories for the Day			

Describe your activity today:

……

……

……

LIFE STYLE WEIGHT MANAGEMENT

DAILY FOOD DAIRY

Date: …………………….

Time you woke up: …………………………………………..

Time you went to bed: …………………………………………

Time	Food/Beverages/Ingredients	Portion/Size	Est. Calories	Feel Full?
	Total Calories for the Day			

Describe your activity today:

………………………………………………………………………………………………………

………………………………………………………………………………………………………

………………………………………………………………………………………………………

DAILY FOOD DAIRY

Date: …………………….

Time you woke up: ………………………………………..

Time you went to bed: …………………………………….

Please list the brand names, ingredients and portion of each food you eat daily.

Time	Food/Beverages/Ingredients	Portion/Size	Est. Calories	Feel Full?
	Total Calories for the Day			

Describe your activity today:

………

………

………

LIFE STYLE WEIGHT MANAGEMENT

DAILY FOOD DAIRY

Date: …………………….

Time you woke up: …………………………………………….

Time you went to bed: ………………………………………………

Time	Food/Beverages/Ingredients	Portion/Size	Est. Calories	Feel Full?
	Total Calories for the Day			

Describe your activity today:

………

………

………

DAILY FOOD DAIRY

Date: …………………….

Time you woke up: ………………………………………..

Time you went to bed: …………………………………………

Please list the brand names, ingredients and portion of each food you eat daily.

Time	Food/Beverages/Ingredients	Portion/Size	Est. Calories	Feel Full?
	Total Calories for the Day			

Describe your activity today:

………

………

……………………………………………………………………………………………………

LIFE STYLE WEIGHT MANAGEMENT

DAILY FOOD DAIRY

Date: ....

Time you woke up: ....

Time you went to bed: ....

Time	Food/Beverages/Ingredients	Portion/Size	Est. Calories	Feel Full?
	Total Calories for the Day			

Describe your activity today:

....

....

....

LIFE STYLE WEIGHT MANAGEMENT

DAILY FOOD DAIRY

Date: …………………

Time you woke up: ………………………………………..

Time you went to bed: ……………………………………………

Time	Food/Beverages/Ingredients	Portion/Size	Est. Calories	Feel Full?
	Total Calories for the Day			

Describe your activity today:

………

………

………

LIFE STYLE WEIGHT MANAGEMENT

DAILY FOOD DAIRY

Date: ……………………

Time you woke up: …………………………………….

Time you went to bed: ……………………………………….

Please list the brand names, ingredients and portion of each food you eat daily.

Time	Food/Beverages/Ingredients	Portion/Size	Est. Calories	Feel Full?
	Total Calories for the Day			

Describe your activity today:

………

………

………

DAILY FOOD DAIRY

Date: …………………….

Time you woke up: ……………………………………………..

Time you went to bed: ………………………………………….

Please list the brand names, ingredients and portion of each food you eat daily.

Time	Food/Beverages/Ingredients	Portion/Size	Est. Calories	Feel Full?
	Total Calories for the Day			

Describe your activity today:

……

……

……

DAILY FOOD DAIRY

Date: …………………….

Time you woke up: ………………………………………………….

Time you went to bed: ………………………………………………….

Please list the brand names, ingredients and portion of each food you eat daily.

Time	Food/Beverages/Ingredients	Portion/Size	Est. Calories	Feel Full?
	Total Calories for the Day			

Describe your activity today:

………………………………………………………………………………………………………

………………………………………………………………………………………………………

………………………………………………………………………………………………………

LIFE STYLE WEIGHT MANAGEMENT

DAILY FOOD DAIRY

Date: …………………….

Time you woke up: …………………………………………..

Time you went to bed: ………………………………………….

Time	Food/Beverages/Ingredients	Portion/Size	Est. Calories	Feel Full?
	Total Calories for the Day			

Describe your activity today:

………

………

………

LIFE STYLE WEIGHT MANAGEMENT

DAILY FOOD DAIRY

Date: ………………….

Time you woke up: ………………………………………….

Time you went to bed: ………………………………………….

Time	Food/Beverages/Ingredients	Portion/Size	Est. Calories	Feel Full?
	Total Calories for the Day			

Describe your activity today:

………………………………………………………………………………………………

………………………………………………………………………………………………

………………………………………………………………………………………………

DAILY FOOD DAIRY

Date: …………………….

Time you woke up: …………………………………………..

Time you went to bed: ……………………………………………

Please list the brand names, ingredients and portion of each food you eat daily.

Time	Food/Beverages/Ingredients	Portion/Size	Est. Calories	Feel Full?
	Total Calories for the Day			

Describe your activity today:

………

………

……………………………………………………………………………………………………

LIFE STYLE WEIGHT MANAGEMENT

DAILY FOOD DAIRY

Date: …………………….

Time you woke up: ………………………………………..

Time you went to bed: ……………………………………………

Time	Food/Beverages/Ingredients	Portion/Size	Est. Calories	Feel Full?
	Total Calories for the Day			

Describe your activity today:

……

……

……

LIFE STYLE WEIGHT MANAGEMENT

DAILY FOOD DAIRY

Date: …………………….

Time you woke up: ………………………………………………..

Time you went to bed: …………………………………………….

Please list the brand names, ingredients and portion of each food you eat daily.

Time	Food/Beverages/Ingredients	Portion/Size	Est. Calories	Feel Full?
	Total Calories for the Day			

Describe your activity today:

………

………

………

LIFE STYLE WEIGHT MANAGEMENT

DAILY FOOD DAIRY

Date: …………………….

Time you woke up: ……………………………………………..

Time you went to bed: ……………………………………………

Please list the brand names, ingredients and portion of each food you eat daily.

Time	Food/Beverages/Ingredients	Portion/Size	Est. Calories	Feel Full?
	Total Calories for the Day			

Describe your activity today:

………

………

………

LIFE STYLE WEIGHT MANAGEMENT

DAILY FOOD DAIRY

Date: …………………….

Time you woke up: ………………………………………………..

Time you went to bed: ………………………………………………

Please list the brand names, ingredients and portion of each food you eat daily.

Time	Food/Beverages/Ingredients	Portion/Size	Est. Calories	Feel Full?
	Total Calories for the Day			

Describe your activity today:

……

……

……

LIFE STYLE WEIGHT MANAGEMENT

DAILY FOOD DAIRY

Date: …………………….

Time you woke up: …………………………………………..

Time you went to bed: …………………………………………

Time	Food/Beverages/Ingredients	Portion/Size	Est. Calories	Feel Full?
	Total Calories for the Day			

Describe your activity today:

……………………………………………………………………………………………………

……………………………………………………………………………………………………

……………………………………………………………………………………………………

LIFE STYLE WEIGHT MANAGEMENT

DAILY FOOD DAIRY

Date: …………………….

Time you woke up: …………………………………………..

Time you went to bed: ………………………………………….

Please list the brand names, ingredients and portion of each food you eat daily.

Time	Food/Beverages/Ingredients	Portion/Size	Est. Calories	Feel Full?
	Total Calories for the Day			

Describe your activity today:

……

……

……

DAILY FOOD DAIRY

Date: …………………….

Time you woke up: ………………………………………….

Time you went to bed: …………………………………………….

Please list the brand names, ingredients and portion of each food you eat daily.

Time	Food/Beverages/Ingredients	Portion/Size	Est. Calories	Feel Full?
	Total Calories for the Day			

Describe your activity today:

………

………

………

LIFE STYLE WEIGHT MANAGEMENT

DAILY FOOD DAIRY

Date: …………………….

Time you woke up: ………………………………………..

Time you went to bed: …………………………………………

Please list the brand names, ingredients and portion of each food you eat daily.

Time	Food/Beverages/Ingredients	Portion/Size	Est. Calories	Feel Full?
	Total Calories for the Day			

Describe your activity today:

………

………

……………………………………………………………………………

LIFE STYLE WEIGHT MANAGEMENT

DAILY FOOD DAIRY

Date: …………………..

Time you woke up: ………………………………………….

Time you went to bed: …………………………………………

Please list the brand names, ingredients and portion of each food you eat daily.

Time	Food/Beverages/Ingredients	Portion/Size	Est. Calories	Feel Full?
	Total Calories for the Day			

Describe your activity today:

……

……

……

LIFE STYLE WEIGHT MANAGEMENT

DAILY FOOD DAIRY

Date: …………………….

Time you woke up: ……………………………………..

Time you went to bed: …………………………………….

Time	Food/Beverages/Ingredients	Portion/Size	Est. Calories	Feel Full?
	Total Calories for the Day			

Describe your activity today:

………………………………………………………………………………………………………

………………………………………………………………………………………………………

………………………………………………………………………………………………………

LIFE STYLE WEIGHT MANAGEMENT

DAILY FOOD DAIRY

Date: …………………….

Time you woke up: ……………………………………..

Time you went to bed: ………………………………………

Time	Food/Beverages/Ingredients	Portion/Size	Est. Calories	Feel Full?
	Total Calories for the Day			

Describe your activity today:

………

………

………

LIFE STYLE WEIGHT MANAGEMENT

DAILY FOOD DAIRY

Date: …………………….

Time you woke up: ………………………………………………..

Time you went to bed: ……………………………………………

Please list the brand names, ingredients and portion of each food you eat daily.

Time	Food/Beverages/Ingredients	Portion/Size	Est. Calories	Feel Full?
	Total Calories for the Day			

Describe your activity today:

……

……

……